## A MESSAGE TO THE READER

Sir/Madam

Greetings in the Mighty Name of our LORD and SAVIOR, JESUS the CHRIST.

I speak to all the people of Earth, since we are a small community connected by the Internet on AMBUSH, the CURE for HIV/AIDS. In 2002 I was divinely given Ambush for ALL OF US.

The LORD GOD JAHOVA , Creator of Heaven and Earth has commanded me to tell you that He EXISTS, and HE has heard our many prayers and has answered us , but it is up to us to receive AMBUSH, the CURE for HIV/AIDS.

Father, in the Mighty name of Jesus the Christ, we thank you for your gift of Ambush to all of us and we receive it in Jesus' name......AMEN (let the reader agree with all of us in thanksgiving and receipt by saying aloud...amen)

50 PAGES OF HOPE......the BOOK

This is the year 2014 in an age where everything seems to be going very fast, an era of the text message where every word is shortened and time is of the essence, then kindly allow me to deliver this message of HOPE in 50 PAGES. Biblical HOPE is based on a promise from The LORD GOD JAHOVA. Exodus 15: 26 says,

*"If you diligently heed the voice of the LORD your GOD and do what is right in His sight, give ear to His commandments and keep all His statutes, I will put none of the diseases on you which I have I have brought on the Egyptians for I am the LORD that heals you."*

Again in Psalm 103:2-3 David writes

*Bless the LORD O my soul, and forget not his benefits: Who forgives all our iniquities, Who heals all your diseases.*

The LORD GOD JAHOVA has made a contract with believers to take care of their health and has provided doctors and medicine as is seen in Numbers 21: 8-9, Then the LORD said to Moses,

> "*Make a fiery serpent, and set it on a pole: and it shall be that everyone who is bitten, when he looks at it shall live," So Moses made a bronze serpent, and put it on a pole: and so it was, if a serpent had bitten any one, when he looked at the bronze serpent, he lived.*"

Is that not now the logo of medicine, a snake or serpent wrapped around a pole? Do not all medicines come from the Earth?

To all who are infected with HIV, affected by HIV and ALL OF US, we greet you in the Mighty Name of or LORD and Savior, JESUS the CHRIST. We bring a message of HOPE from The Kingdom of Heaven that the LORD GOD JAHOVA has given us AMBUSH, the CURE for HIV/AIDS.

It is April 22, 2002 and I am a 49 year old Pharmacist working in the Hospital systems in Miami, Florida. For the past 5 years I have been working two and sometimes three jobs at the same time. I had this great idea that I should quickly pay off all my debts and move to Tallahassee, Florida. I would then buy a small farm in a hilly area that I had once driven by. There it would be close enough to the hospitals in Tallahassee where I would work part-time, maybe, and quietly retire into a lazy life forever.......

I had been dreaming of this lazy life style for about six months and was beginning to make plans to drive up to Tallahassee on my next day off. The problem was that I had been working seven days per week and had locked myself into such a position that it was hard to arrange a few days off, neither did I want to because I would loose the revenue so there was this struggle as to when to leave Miami but in the meantime I worked sixteen hours per day for many days in the week.

With these long hours, I was deprived of sleep and pretended to be in school and I kept telling myself that it was all a dream and I would soon wake up as soon as I enough money to leave Miami and at least semi retire at age 50, make enough to merely exist. But what about the kids? Would the family move?

There were serious struggles and I had this feeling that I had to leave Miami but I could not figure out how or when it would happen, but I knew it would happen. I had to work ever other weekend on the regular full time job and had slowly began cutting back on the other weekend so I could catch up on sleep. I had worked Sunday and was due for work on Monday from 3pm to 11.30 pm, but had awoken by 10 am. At about 1 pm I laid in the bed to rest an hour before getting ready for work.

I am not sure if I dozed off and if so for how long when I had an experience, a dream or a vision I am not really sure. Yet I have been having dreams and visions since I was a child, but this one was so real, so different, so pronounced that I do not think I will ever forget it.

## A VISION FROM THE ANGEL GABRIEL

My second life began on April 22, 2002, when I had just gone to bed. I was not asleep but semiconscious when an angel appeared at the doorway, standing on the penultimate step.

Gabriel: "I am here to give you the CURE for Aids"

Vernon: "Right…….there is no CURE for Aids!"

Gabriel: "Do you believe that I am an Angel?

First, I thought that this Being was joking, or that I was dreaming so I turned to get a good look at the Angel. He was wearing a white robe, he had a tan complexion and I was only viewing him from his right side. He was very serious and had a stern look ...like that of my mother when I am misbehaving.

Vernon: "Yes....."

Then I paused and asked...

Vernon: "What is it?"

Then Gabriel took me outside in the Spirit and showed me the 'PALM' plant, certain specie that is commonly grown in Miami and in tropical regions of the world.

Gabriel: "It is in this."

Vernon: "But, we (meaning the scientific community) have studied this plant and there is nothing in it!"

Gabriel: "Since you (meaning man) have studied it, We (meaning the Kingdom of Heaven) have put it in."

Vernon: "How do we get it out?"

Gabriel: "Take a piece of palm (about such and such long, boil it) then drink it three times daily for 21days (then there was a long pause) and it is to be FREE"

Vernon: "Why me?"

Gabriel: "Why not you?"

Vernon:"You got me there….. (Pause)...do you realize how this is going to change my lifestyle?"

Gabriel: "Yes… (Now he turned and looked me straight in the eyes with the sweetest, kindest and gentlest smile)...let me show you."

Then he took me to the window and showed me hundreds of TV station mobile units lining all four streets that bordered the house.

Then Gabriel left and I was now exited, fearful, in a state of shock and generally very unsettled. I thought I had a bad dream and it would soon be forgotten but something deep inside me said I was to read all the angel accounts in the Bible. I did and every time I read them, something happened to me on the inside like a very unsettled feeling that urged me to go on.

For the next several months, I pondered what was happening. I tried to make sense of what I had been told. Was it true? Who would believe me? Who should I tell? What was I supposed to do with piece of information? The questions kept rolling in my head and I was as happy as I was sad and all my emotions were rolled into a ball of confusion with as many questions and not really having any avenue to disseminate this precious piece of information.

It was 2002 and HIV/AIDS had been ravishing the world since 1980 and the scientific community was giving the world many different tales that the cure or a vaccine was right around the corner. As a pharmacist like the rest of the health care community we were all required to have a certain amount of continuing education credits on the latest information on HIV.

What was I supposed to do with this information that I had received from the Kingdom of

Heaven? I sent it to a number of research institutions by way of email and the one that answered me wanted to know how I came into this information and if it in fact worked. This was a frustrating experience considering that here I was divinely given the CURE for HIV/AIDS and I was trying to give it to the Scientific Researchers and nobody would even answer me.

After the first months of trying to give this information to anybody who would or could use it and nobody seemed to care or believe me I became frustrated. So on the last Sunday in September during the prayer session at church I asked The LORD GOD JAHOVA,

"What am I to do with the information?"

The same angel answered and said,

"Go to Evangelist (such and such), and when your name is Reverend Vernon Palmer Rph. then people will listen to you because I want the CURE to come through my Church".

I can still remember the command and was just beginning to process what was happening realizing that the situation was true, real and serious. The happy feel that I had spoken to an angel had now changed into a serious reality that my life was about to change radically and fears of the unknown started to creep into my mind.  From that Sunday, I felt like I was carrying the weight of the world on my head until I found the Evangelist two weeks later at

Universal Deliverance Church where a convention that was in progress. There I cried my heart out to her not knowing then that I was under the anointing of the Holy Spirit since I had grown up in the Anglican Church, later attended a Catholic Church and nothing was ever said about the anointing power of the Holy Spirit. Outside the church, she touched my belly and I expelled raw emotions as to the task ahead with a deep gut feeling that the Lord wanted me to take this CURE to the world.  What a task? Could I do it?

I sent my dreams to many researchers and scientists in the field of HIV research and had gotten no answers least anything favorable so I was beginning to feel that I was the One that The Lord wanted to carry this to the world. The next step was to start working on it and The Lord would help me so it is now March 2, 2003 and I went out and obtained a piece of the Palm plant. I was surprised to find that it was tough and barky. I cut a few pieces and put it on the stove with some water to boil. I had seen in a vision that I had two bottles of the boiled substance and one had more crystals than the other.

In reality, I prepared it as I had seen in the vision but decided to send one bottle to a lab for testing, thinking that whatever was in one would be in the other. So I boiled it, poured it in a Pyrex bottle, a dark brown liquid that started to separate to a white powder at the bottom when cooled. When shaken, it became a brown liquid which I took to a lab in Miami. The old scientist ran a number of tests starting with poisons or any harmful substance known to man and he found none. He also searched for any new substance but none were then found.

I got some more plant materials, cut it up, boiled it but found nothing of substance in the pot but there was a 'gel' on the cover that hardened after a few days to form a small crystal. I was beginning to really work on the project so I got an old tree, cut two pieces of about six inches and took them to the kitchen. As I started to prepare them, there was a very strong smell of 'Jamaican curry' around the plant material and no one was cooking. I boiled the piece which produced a lot of gel and I prayed for lots of crystals which contained the active ingredient of Ambush, the CURE for AIDS.

It is March 4, 2003 and I left the store at 2:30pm and was on my way home when I was overcome by the Holy Spirit who told me that tomorrow, Ash Wednesday I am to fast for forty days. With tears of the anointing in my eyes I agreed thinking that if Jesus did it without food, then I could do it with food after 6 pm. At 3:30 pm I took the second sample to the lab and that day they found 'crystals' between the fibers. Later I also found crystals under the microscope at 200 magnification along with oil droplets.

I had by April 2003, did an extensive list of tests and found no poisonous substance, since I am living in America and the first question is to the harmful effects of this new substance.

My next plan was to find someone who is HIV positive to give it a try and see if it worked as the Angel had said but let us first look at the Laws.

## LAWS OF CONFIDENTIALITY

Confidentiality means that personal information is kept private, and may not be shared without the persons' permission. The confidentiality of a person's HIV status is important because people with HIV and AIDS face discrimination when other people find out that they have HIV. People will only get tested for HIV if they know that their HIV status will be kept quiet.

The United State of America is a country of Laws. There are multiple layers of Laws, each covering and governing the conduct of every aspect of life and are all vigorously enforced so the common man thinks and knows about his rights.

Federal and State Laws require that a persons' HIV status be kept confidential. The Health Insurance Portability and Accountability Act (known as HIPAA) is the federal law that protects the privacy of a person's health information. The Confidentiality of HIV-Related Information Acts say that a health care provider or social service provider cannot share HIV test results without written permission but with its exceptions.

I have been asked many times who are the people that we have sent or given Ambush to as a means of ascertaining whether it works or not. These questions are never answered because if I told you that I sent Ambush to Charles Albert Palmer of Warsop, Trelawny, then every

Charles Palmer will sue me for breach of the Confidentiality Laws by telling you that he got Ambush. The reasoning is that since Ambush CURES HIV/AIDS, then, if I sent it, it would be because Charles Palmer is HIV positive thus divulging his status.

I am often asked how many people have I given Ambush and the answer is that I do not and will never know. At the clinic I was running in Miami, I used to ask for names and addresses as required by other Laws when medicaments are given out and I had ten names on a page and had 40 pages. I was reading 2 Samuel Chapter 24 where the anger of the LORD was kindled against Israel and He caused David to take a census of Israel and Judah. This census or numbering of the people gave the

LORD permission to release wrath on the people. In this situation, I am not permitted to number His people on His project so after 12 years of giving and sending Ambush, I have no idea as to how many people have received Ambush but only pray that many more had received it.

On the other hand I know there are millions of HIV positive people who are waiting and praying that a CURE be found, if not for them but for their children and grand children. This is a book of HOPE to say yes, there is a CURE and even if it does not come to fruition in your lifetime, you heard that it will be available for the next generation.

This is why the Kingdom of Heaven gave me the title 50 PAGES of HOPE, to tell the waiting world that

He sent Ambush since 2002 and we the body of Christ have not yet received it. The reason for this HOPE is that people who have taken Ambush are coming up HIV NEGATIVE after 5 months and it will only be a matter of time before Ambush will become a household name in ONE DAY.

Jesus was speaking to all of us in John 11: 40 when He said,

*"Did I not say to you that if you would believe, you would see the glory of GOD?"*

You have to believe first and then see, Jesus was not joking, He is serious at all times. Too often the phrase 'seeing is believing' is heard in the body of Christ. If you can see it, then it is there and no need to believe. It is in believing that the body of Christ brings into being something that is not yet there in the physical. So the message here is one of HOPE so that when we believe, it gives the Almighty permission to do mighty works here in the earth.

THE FIRST PERSON TO TRY AMBUSH.

It was not very hard to find to find a person in Miami that was willing to try Ambush since this has always been a project run by The Kingdom of Heaven. I told a few of my friends and the word went around 'quietly' as if it is such a hush that nobody wanted to speak about the subject due to its stigma.

In a dream the LORD shows me one of my friends who was dying of AIDS. I saw his mother in the dream and she said that I was to reconcile with her son Ted (name changed) because he did not have long to live. I had seen Ted a few months earlier and he was a healthy looking man of about 40 years old working long days as we all did as Jamaicans in Miami.

So I went to his house and I was shocked to see Ted. He was very sick, and could not get out of bed without assistance. He had lost half his body mass and was having diarrhea, with a body that had dropped from 200 to about 125 pounds.

In sickness or times of eminent death, all squabbling are forgiven and forgotten since we had more pressing issues at hand. So I told him about Ambush and asked him if he was willing to try it. He was eager and thankful that he was being remembered with real help since the anti diarrheal medicines were not seem to be working.

I went home and prepared the first batch of Ambush, and since he had no body mass, I made some cornmeal porridge and added some vegetable oil which is one remedy for malnutrition. I gave him the first dose that day since I was boiling the green plant and it easily yielded its medicine. The dose was 60 ml three times daily for 21 days. By day number 3 Ted was strong enough to go the bathroom by himself. The diarrhea had stopped and within the week he was outside walking. I took him to Jackson Medical Center and there he was tested positive for HIV.

In three weeks, Ted had improver to the point he could go back to work and I had a lot of work to do to tell and convince the world of what the Kingdom of Heaven was doing on Earth. Thank you Jesus for Ambush!

THE SCIENCE OF AMBUSH

WHAT is a CURE???

Dictionaries define a CURE as the restoration of health or a recovery from a disease. If a CURE then the body should be restored to its original form and no harmful aftereffects.

WHAT is AMBUSH???

In researching Ambush for the past 12 years I can safely say that it is a substance that kills the virus and thereby allows the body to return to its original state. To clarify this statement, it depends on the age and health of the person. If the person is young say less than 40 years old then the body is able to return to a healthy position. If the person is older in their 50"s, then other health issues may have arisen because of the HIV infection. So a course of Ambush would CURE the HIV but the other issues may linger. Ambush is taken by mouth into the body so we could start the discussion as to what happens in the gastrointestinal tract GI which starts at the mouth and ends in the rectum.

The same kinds of cells that are found in the mouth are also found as the lining for the GI track with differences depending on their functions at that particular area. Drugs such as ARV's are absorbed from the stomach to the intestines into the blood stream. If the stomach lining is infected with HIV, then it is difficult to get a certain blood level to flow back into the stomach to effect change in the virus.

EFFECTS OF AMBUSH IN THE MOUTH.

Digestion and absorption starts in the mouth so let us look at what happens in the mouth. The scientific community says that you cannot catch HIV from saliva, but if a person infected with HIV spits on a Police officer, he is charged with assault with a deadly weapon, or as a Bio-terrorist. So I am saying that HIV can be transmitted through saliva. When Ambush is taken, it kills the viruses that are in the mouth lining and this causes the person to have a dry mouth with a change of taste.

## DADE COUNTY SCHOOL

I wrestled with the question as to whether or not a person could catch HIV from saliva and The LORD GOD JAHOVA showed me in a vision a school in Dade County which had about 1600 kids with ages from about 7 or 8 years old to about 14 to 16. I did not check the true details because the revelation was so frightening when He said to me,

"All the kids in that school are HIV positive."

So I said to the LORD,

"Show me because those little kids are not having sex."

Then the LORD took me in the Spirit into the school on a hot afternoon to the water cooler. There were a large number of kids waiting to drink from the cooler. The water from the cooler should squirt about 4to 6 inches but only came up an inch the most so all the kids sucked on the faucet. A kid would buy a soda from the machine and all four of his friends were given a sip.

If you research HIV in kids, there is not too much because the kids are not being tested. At the same time, they are growing and their growth hormones are able to keep the virus in check and so the kids do not get sick. The problem arises when they have stopped growing and the virus decides to explode.

At this same time I went to see Ted at his workshop and I saw his 15 year old son take a sip from his soda and gave it back to Ted. The LORD then showed me how the re-infection could have taken place. If you are shocked to read this, then think of how I was when I was there seeing it happen and hearing the voice of the Almighty!

I can write this because I have seen Ambush work and I know that the LORD GOD JAHOVA has given us the CURE. So I speak the truth. This book is called 50 PAGES of HOPE to give HOPE to the millions of people in the World who are infected with HIV and all the rest of us.

Let us give a shout of thanks and praise to the MOST HIGH JAHOVA for his mercy, goodness and love for his created beings that he has answered the prayers of millions of people who have been praying for such a moment as this. In the Book of

Genesis, chapter 19, the LORD rained down fire and brimstone on the inhabitants of Sodom and Gomorrah because of their deeds. Let us look deeper into a story of love and compassion and you ask, "How is that so?"

A piece of brimstone is 99% Sulfur and it burns at a temperature of 3000 degrees to give off sulfur dioxide and sulfur trioxide gas which when inhaled produces sulfuric acid in the lungs which kills the person in minutes of not being able to breathe. So the inhabitants would have died a relatively quick death. Most people would have passed out after inhaling the fumes so their death would be almost painless. So even in destruction, the LORD is merciful and did not allow the inhabitants to suffer.  How much more his compassion to those all over  the earth that have become infected through blood transfusion, close contact, needle stick or even a mosquito bite? Ambush is here to give HOPE.

The Kingdom of Heaven has shown me in a number of steps how to isolate the active ingredient from the plant and commercially produce it. This is in itself HOPE because I have isolated the active ingredient and sent it to a government agency and I have yet to receive a reply. This is HOPE because people have been cured and we only need one person to go public with their results and the world will hear in one day.

ACTION of AMBUSH ON THE GI TRACK

It is known that late stage AIDS people posse a high level of virus in the GUT which should include the entire GI tract from stomach to rectum. Here the virus is found in the lining and this is difficult to treat with ARV's because these are the areas needed by the ARV's to enter the blood supply. There is not a high enough blood level returning back to the stomach lining hence the virus remains in high concentration and kills the stomach lining. This causes the person's appetite to decrease which causes a spiraling downhill of the body.

When Ambush is taken as a liquid, it is slightly basic and forms a stable compound in the acidic stomach. This Ambush compound is close to the stomach lining to exert a 'natural radioactivity' effect which kills the virus in the stomach. Here the entire midsection feels very warm and sometimes feverish. The infected stomach and GI lining with the dead areas is then passed out as a grey to black slime in the stool. This usually happens on about day 4 while on a 21 day course of 60 ml, three times daily, wherein the person has a large bowel movement.

After the bowel movement, the person becomes extremely hungry and eats 2 to 3 times a normal serving. Here I usually recommend cornmeal porridge with butter or vegetable oil as prevention against malnutrition and a daily multivitamin.

By day 10, the GI track is recovering and the person eats normally.

Other people have reported that they will have the urge to defecate but only to pass out a grey to dark brown slime which is the walls of the GI track. These are areas that were infected with HIV that are being replaced.

Smokers told me that after a few days on Ambush they can feel when the lining of their throat peels from its place and falls as a big glob down their throat leaving an empty clean feeling at the back of their throat which allows them to breathe much easier.

AMBUSH WORKS like
RADIOIMMUNOTHERAPY

Ambush kills the virus by a
process that closely resembles
Radioimmunotherapy, a process that
is being researched at the Albert
Einstein College of Medicine in the
Bronx, New York. Here the
researchers lower the viral load to
undetectable using ARV's and then
try to kill the rest of virus with a
steady dose of radiation. It is not
clear as to their method of
application or the version used to
treat leukemia but they complain of
the 'latent cells' which make HIV a
challenge. If they used 10 units of
radiation, this would not be able to
penetrate all the body tissues for a
long enough period of time to kill all
the viruses in the body using a

machine. They would need an agent with one unit of radiation that is able to be introduced in the blood that exerts the radioactive properties which kill the virus in every organ in the body for a long enough period of time.

In the case of Ambush, it delivers a steady dose of 'natural radiation' because the active ingredient is an isotope of uranium that is not fully metabolized but excreted virtually unchanged in the urine, stool and skin. When in contact with the virus in the blood, it causes the viral envelope to rupture and the white blood cells mop up the viral particles. The virus that hides in the tendons and the lymph system are killed by this 'natural radiation' process and excreted.

In researching how Ambush worked, the LORD in a vision showed me that a person on Ambush would 'glow' when a chest x-ray was done. So while working at a hospital in Miami I had a person who was on Ambush for about 5 days do a chest x-ray and there was a fuzzed outline on the film when compared to another where the person was not on Ambush. Other x-ray experiments were done on different mediums such as an empty bottle, one with water and another with Ambush to see the fuzz around the bottle with Ambush.

Similar experiments were done by placing a Geiger Counter on and near the container of Ambush and no motion or deflection was noted which would indicate that body heat was the necessary catalyst.

In a discussion with The LORD, He said the amount of radiation in a 21 day treatment was similar to that of one chest x-ray and was safe for pregnant women.

The cells of the vaginal walls are similar to those of the GI track but with different functions. Here the virus behaves much the same way as it does in the GI track. It sticks to the epithelial lining and causes areas to die.

When Ambush is taken by females, it acts similar to the GI track and kills the viruses that are in the vaginal cell walls. This tissue is then expelled as mucus of varying colors. If she takes Ambush during her menstrual cycle then she should experience a heavier than normal blood flow with clumps of vaginal wall tissue being expelled. Women that take Ambush outside the cycle report that there is sometimes a discharge of mucus. The degree or severity of the discharge seems to reflect the amount of virus in the body.

AMBUSH CURES HIV/AIDS....EFFECTS
on the SKIN

The skin is the largest organ of
the body with many different
functions such as the covering for the
entire body which protects against
heat, light, injury and infection. It also
regulates body temperature, stores
water, fat and other substances. One
of its main functions is in the
excretion of waste matter in the form
of sweat which also acts as body
cooling. The skin is sensitive to touch
and is an organ of beauty.

The skin of an HIV infected
person is a nightmare to
dermatologist because of the
interaction between the immune
system and the HIV which causes
itchy skin rashes. There are then skin
problems caused by infections which

are generally rashes, eczemas, sores or boils. Let us not forget skin conditions caused by the side effects of drugs and particularly those taken in the treatment of HIV/AIDS, where the list of skin conditions seem more deadly and frightening than the disease.

When Ambush kills the virus the viral particles are excreted in the urine, stool and through the skin. Depending on the age of the person and how long he has been infected, there are many changes to the skin. In dark skinned people, it seems that the virus attaches itself to the melanin on the face and causes darker patches in the face which generally lightens up after the first week of Ambush. In light skinned people, the infection usually causes the skin to be dry and scaly. This is again reversed after a week on Ambush.

Since the dead viral particles are excreted through the skin, then there is sometimes a rash that develops when a person starts Ambush. This is because the skin is not healthy and the particles are trapped in the skin. To clear these trapped particles, the LORD showed me that the people are to use peanut oil and rub the entire body after bathing. They are then to wait a few minutes so that the oil will dry into the skin. This means the oil penetrates the skin and leaves no oil on the skin but dry to the touch.

The oil then picks up the viral particles and deposits them into the blood stream and is later passed out in the stool where the fat droplets may be seen in the toilet.

After about 2 weeks of such treatment, the unhealthy skin clears up, is renewed, looks and feels like that of a child and is now healthy.

We know that the immune system kills some of the virus in the body, hence the positive antibodies and they are excreted through the skin. But what if there are sores on the body? These sore may not heal in a 21 day treatment as this dose was given for those who have unbroken skin.

When I am approached for Ambush, I now inquire if the person has any cuts, sores, operations or torn muscles or ligaments. This is because this is an area where the virus hides and so the LORD showed me over time to adjust the dosage for these cases. In hiding, the virus forms a cocoon or tight knit ball of itself. It uses a layer virus to cover one virus then another layer of virus to cover the first layer. So it puts layer upon layer to spin a unit that is hard to penetrate with ARV's. The idea is that if a substance is able to kill the first outer layer, then there are thousands more that will not be penetrated. The virus then sits and waits until the threat has passed and the untouched layers are back in business. In a sore are thousands of cocoons which cause resistance to ARV's. Here the ARV's pass in the blood stream and are not in high enough blood levels to affect the cocoons.

My first encounter with 'viral cocoons' was with Mr. Lab at the hospital. We had become friends so that I could access some results that were outside the chart. The LORD told me to tell him to do a Western blot test on himself since the LORD wanted to use him in the Ambush Project. (Western blot test is the confirmatory test for HIV) He laughed and said that it was not possible for him to be infected with HIV because of his years of precaution and knowledge of microbes. If the LORD had told me and it was found to be true, then he would have to throw out all his belief systems and he was not about to do that.

Two months later he came to the Pharmacy and said he was going to be operated on to remove his appendix. I told him to remember his pre-existing condition and he laughed and said I was "crazy". So he was operated on the following week and all seemed well until he was sent to Recovery Room where he spiked a temperature and ended up in the Intensive Care Unit for two weeks. The medical staff was busy trying to find out what caused this downhill slide in an ordinary healthy 50 year old male. He was discharged to the floor for another week before going home. While on the floor, I went to review his chart but someone had thinned the chart and it only had a mere 10 pages as opposed to the 100 that I was expecting.

A month later, he came back to work and at lunch, he asked me what had happened and why was he now feeling worst than before. The LORD showed me in a vision that since he was a fat man, the top layer of skin healed but the fat layer or hypodermis had not healed but had formed pockets of HIV which caused the area not to heal but to attract other microbes and this caused is down hill slide.

My second example is that of Pastor Memphis who was directed to me by the Kingdom of Heaven and he came and received one supply of Ambush so I gave him a few more, just in case. In his first few days of Ambush he experienced great changes with emphasis that a lot of his energy had returned and in a few weeks his eating ability was back and so I thought all would be well and we were in the waiting period of 5

months when he would serorevert to
HIV negative. The time came and he
said he was not quite well and was
not sure what was happening. So I
took his case to the Kingdom of
Heaven in prayer. The LORD said I
was to ask him if he had and sores or
cuts on the body. I was shocked when
he sent me a picture of a sore that
was on the private in the folds of an
uncircumcised penis. I asked how
long has it been there and I was told
it has been there for more than a
year since the last outbreak of HPV.

Then the LORD gave me a new
dose that would kill the viral cocoons
in sores as 5 Grams daily for 10 days
or until the sore was healed. So many
of our peoples have sore that ooze
cocoons of HIV and expensive
treatments at a wound care clinic

does a good job of covering the wound, only to have it break out after the treatment has stopped. Now we have been given the CURE to the sores in people with HIV, we give all thanks and praised to the MOST HIGH JAHOVA.

## SOME EFFECTS and SIDE EFFECTS of AMBUSH

### (1) Headaches

All drugs have side effects which are other effects than those intended as the purpose of that drug. Since Ambush is a drug, it too has negative and positive side effects. In the last 12 years of giving out Ambush, the most common side effect is that of headache. One gentleman in Miami complained of severe headache on the fifth day of treatment and since I have no earthly consultations, I asked the Kingdom of Heaven. Headaches result when there is no more live virus to be killed so the Kingdom has built in a natural stopping point. I have found that most HIV persons who take Ambush will experience a headache at about day 17 but it is mild and will last an hour and then go away until the next dose.

The persons with sores do not seem to experience headaches at the dose of 10 days supply daily for 10 or more days. There is Miss Wheelchair who in not able to walk because the myelin sheath covering the spine has been eroded and now there are pockets of virus in the cocoons that are in the spaces of her spinal column. Even after the first 10 days she has not had a headache but the smell of Ambush being prepared to a person who is HIV free, gives them a headache. Her viral load on 5/6/14 was 441,476 but DROPPED on 6/20/14 to 226,900 and that is HOPE, even to the unbelieving scientific community at Johns Hopkins in Maryland.

(2) Increased Libido

One of the first most noted effects in male on Ambush is that there is an added amount of erections that start at about day 5. For the women, the same increase in libido starting around day 7 which causes weak willed individuals to go back to the same behavior that maybe got then infected in the first place.

On examination as to the reason we looked at the prostate, and testicles to find that the level of virus in the blood may be at an undetectable level but a blood sample from the prostate shows a high viral load. This is because the virus sits in the prostate where there is a healthy supply of rich blood and causes the decrease in the production of testosterone, the hormone that is necessary for erections. The medical community tries to overcome this by giving testosterone supplements.

Similarly in women, testosterone is produced in the ovaries which are well served with rich blood supplies. Here again HIV causes a drop in this hormone so there is little to no urge for sexual activities. What I have said is well documented but there is good news.

Ambush kills the virus that is primarily in the blood in about 7 days, which frees up the testosterone producing mechanism. When this restarts, it sends large amounts of testosterone into the blood stream and the male body reacts with erections similar to those of adolescence. Similar situation happened to the women who were comfortable with the subject to discuss it with me.

## (3) SKIN COLOR and CHANGES.

As indicated earlier, there are some connections with the coloration of a person's skin that is HIV positive and in most case seem to increase the melanin which is responsible for the skin color and leaves it looking as if there is an extra layer of skin on the person. When Ambush is taken the reverse can be seen where the skin color gradually lightens in the first week and the changes continue until the skin goes back to its natural color.

There is therefore HOPE for the people who are HIV positive and are experiencing some or all the problems of living with HIV. The message from the LORD GOD JAHOVA is that there is a CURE for HIV that He has given us since 2002 but we have not accepted it yet neither have we accepted that the Kingdom of Heaven rules the kingdoms of men on the Earth.

## (4) BODY HEAT

When Ambush is taken, the person generally feels an increase in the body temperature. This is especially true for the trunk area which is from the neck down to the knees while the hands and legs remain cool.

AMBUSH CURES
HIV/AIDS....Effects on the Brain

It has been well documented and researched that HIV enters the brain and causes such cognitive problems such as HIV related dementias and milder problems such as trouble focusing and remembering things. HIV is believed to hide in the brain after it disrupts the blood brain barrier to speed brain and body aging by 15 to 17 years. It causes malfunctions of the brain by killing brain cells and preventing stem cells from maturing into adult brain cells. A few symptoms of neurocognitive disorders include:

Confusion

Thinking that is foggy and not clear

Difficulty finding words

Difficulty with fine motor skills such as trying to write legibly

Loss of long and short term memory, trouble with names or dates

Diminished capacity to plan and process problem solving

Lack of motivation and do not seem to care

Personality changes

Difficulty of multitasking or doing two or more things at the same time.

HIV hides in the synapse of the nervous system and for simplification there is the dendrites that bring information to the cell and the axon that takes information from the cell.

The area or space between them is where the virus hides and causes the information to be misread or misinterpreted. The LORD gave me a simple analysis. The synapse may be compared to the electric box of a traffic signal and the system is working well. In a piece of metal accidentally falls into the box or junction, then many problems can occur. Shorting out the circuit, it may cause all four lights to be red wherein all the traffic would stop and wonder when is the light going to change. On the other hand, it could cause all four lights to be green and the results would be a disaster.

HIV is a 'hijacker' that invades the cells, use the cell to produce its offspring, then, kills the nerve cell which causes neurological problems.

Brain cells are replaced in a natural process but when they are killed by HIV, they are not replaced which causes dementia and the brain to shrink.

In the brain, HIV is hard to treat because it hides inside the cells 'protected' from the medicines that travel in the blood stream. There is a need for a substance that can effectively kill the virus and not damaging the brain.

Ambush is a drug or medicine that is also able to pass into the brain to kill the virus by a process of 'natural radiation' and not cause brain problems. So Ambush kills the virus but the natural order of cell replacement has been lost. Brain cells that contain memory have been killed and the memory was not transferred to a young or maturing cell so information is lost. Similar to a computer losing the first 90 pages of your book and you have to start from scratch to relearn how to write.

If you bought a new Bentley motor car and one day it does not start, would you take it to 'Larry's auto repairs' on the same street, one block pass the dealership?

The LORD GOD JAHOVA created us, whether you believe it or not, and I asked him what are we to do about the loss of memory? He said that Ambush will CURE the body but He will CURE the mind. He is the only source by which our minds can be renewed. He made us, so he is the original and has all the spare parts and blueprints in Heaven. He is the master programmer and if we come to Him, He will give us the most updated version of a mind program in Christ. Paul the Apostle, writing to the Romans in chapter 12:2 says,

*And do not be conformed to this world, but be transformed by the renewing of your mind, that you may prove what is that good and acceptable and perfect will of GOD.*

You cannot replace the memory in dead and lost brain cell so you have to seek the face of the Creator who is willing, able and waiting to be asked. You need the Holy Spirit to help in the process. This means that you are now being COMPELLED to come to JESUS CHRIST and be 'born again' by the Holy Spirit. If you do not understand this 'born again' and 'compelled to come to

Jesus' then please find a Bible teaching and believing Church for further information.

Please do not get angry with me, I am not preaching a sermon but only His messenger forcefully delivering His message of HOPE with POWER.

STIGMA of HIV/AIDS

Mankind will only overcome the stigma of HIV/AIDS when Ambush, the CURE for HIV/AIDS comes to fruition. AIDS stigma refers to prejudice and discrimination directed at people who are believed to have HIV or AIDS. Stigma may be defined as the shame or disgrace to something regarded as socially unacceptable. Those who feel stigmatizes feel as outcasts and are marked as being different. This stigma is a world wide practice characterized by

Rejection and avoidance of people with HIV/AIDS

Mandatory HIV testing without consent

Violence against persons perceived of being infected with HIV

Quarantine of persons with HIV

The stigma of HIV does not make us true Humans when people are being stoned to death, fires lit around their necks, fired from their jobs, starved or thrown out of where they are living.

In America, the law says that if you are infected with HIV, then you are compelled to tell your sexual partner or could face time in jail. Are we animals which mate for the procreation of the specie?

One HIV activist once asked the questions, What about love? What about family? Where is unity? Where is trust? What about togetherness? Where is the spirit of oneness? How about group survival? The protection of the group from an external threat such as wars and diseases is an integral part of being a human. Have we as humans been reduced to living behind condoms?

Man as a social entity needs the group for strength and support and not to be the social outcast which HIV has made every person. Sociology of man includes such ideas as social class, mobility, religion and sexuality to mention a few aspects. At all levels of human sociology there are interplays between the social structure and the individual. Here the individual needs to feel as part of the whole body of human being and not as some 'damaged goods' to be cast outside the normal sphere of human living.

Humans change the world and we have changed from the horse and buggy to motor vehicles and now airplanes.

In the beginning of the advent of HIV/AIDS, there was no treatment and people died in large numbers. Later the drug AZT, and now we have various inhibitors and their combinations. Is it so hard to believe that the LORD GOD JAHOVA has given us a new drug that will kill the virus that causes AIDS?

During the days when Jesus walked the Earth, there were colonies of lepers and they stayed away from the general population because there was no CURE and it was contagious. But in Matthew 8: 2-3,

And behold a leper came and worshipped him saying, "Lord if you are willing, you can make me clean" Then Jesus put out his hand and touched him saying, "I am willing: be cleansed."

If Jesus the Christ was willing to heal one leper, how much more the millions of us who are infected and the billions who will be? Since He is the same yesterday, today and forever, why is it that the Body of Christ refuses to believer that their millions of prayers have been answered since 2002 when I was divinely given Ambush, the CURE for HIV/AIDS? Are we waiting until it is on TV before it is believed? Or is it because it is not coming from an institution? The kingdom of men loves committee while the Kingdom of Heaven uses one man.

In the Book of Exodus, the LORD GOD JAHOVA chose Moses to lead the Children of Israel out of Egypt and the job was done according to the words of the Almighty. In Numbers chapter 13, the LORD told Moses to send men to spy out the land. Moses sent 12 spies of which 10 brought back a bad report while only 2 brought back a good report. This shows that the majority is not always right and the LORD does not use a committee.

I have spent the last 12 years listening to the commands of the Almighty so that I could receive Ambush, the CURE for HIV/AIDS and yet the Body of Christ refuses to believe what I have been saying. Is it because I am not singing a song with a high note or preaching a well orated sermon? The body of Christ is a diverse people from the preacher who is anointed to preach to the janitor who is anointed to clean floor one in the same body.

The stigma of HIV will only be removed when Ambush comes to fruition and the world sees that there is a GOD in the Kingdom of Heaven. Let us give thanks and praises to the MOST HIGH JAHOVA for the gift of Ambush which gives HOPE to the millions that the LORD has worked it out.

HIV the PRISON

ALL OF US ARE MERE
PRISONERS to some entity or
another. In Ephesians 3:1, Paul the
Apostle describes himself as a
prisoner for Jesus the Christ. So there
are many different kinds of prisons,
the ones with bars such Alkatraz
where you know whether you are in
or out. Prisons without bars include
addictions to drugs, or alcohol, sin,
sickness, disease and HIV/AIDS to
mention a few. The newspaper
stands of our world could read:

Dallas: Dallas man who infects
teen with HIV gets 75 years in prison

Australia: HIV positive predator
who ruined a woman's life by having
unprotected sex with her without

revealing his status will spend just 9 months in jail for his crime.

America: 52 year old man jailed for 2 years for exposing woman

Canada: 17 year old HIV positive teen girl put on probation for exposing 2 male teenagers with unprotected sex.

Australia: Australian court jails HIV positive man for having unprotected sex.

Canada: Man jailed for not telling partners he has HIV...deported.

France: Untested gay man found criminally liable for 2 previous partners HIV infection.

South Africa: Al Jazeera faces protest over HIV positive journalist. A journalist who was HIV positive dismissed after detained in Doha State Prison.

America: 2 men with HIV jailed for nondisclosure to same man

America: Woman stigmatized and facing felony prosecution for being HIV positive.

America: A New York Supreme court judge ruled a man poses a danger to society and must remain in jail even though his sentence is completed. Prosecutor says for infecting more than 12 women.

Most states in the USA and territories have laws that criminalize HIV exposure and failure by the HIV positive person to disclose their status to their sex partners may result in jail time ranging from a few months to life in prison.

Has the world gone mad? Have we as human beings gone crazy? The truth to the defendants of HIV prosecution is that there is no proof as to how the plaintiff contracted the virus. To break this down, if I am alleged or believed to have transmitted HIV to you, when the virus gets into your body, its RNA attaches to your DNA and your hijacked DNA produces HIV copies while the remnants of the virus are discarded by the body. Can anyone prove that they were not bitten by a mosquito that had bitten an HIV infected person? Can anyone prove they were not infected by the sneeze of someone in a crowded elevator?

The scientific community says that you cannot catch HIV from saliva, but if an HIV positive person spits at an officer, they are charged with trying to infect the officer or worst, as a bio-terrorist. These kinds of situations are not exactly fair and thousands have found themselves in deep waters.

The second kinds of prisons are the ones without bars. These seem far worst because these prisons are on the inside of a person infected with HIV and they are a direct result of the stigma. They tend to be depressed with introverted personalities who seem to be hiding because they do not wish anyone to know they are HIV positive. They carry this shame, this loneliness that has driven many HIV infected people to commit suicide. I have met people whom their doctors have instructed then not to even talk about the subject.

In the Book of Acts of the Apostles, chapter 16:25-26, the Apostles were in jail,

*But at midnight Paul and Silas were praying and singing hymns to GOD, and the prisoners were listening to them. Suddenly there was a great earthquake, so that the foundations of the prison were shaken: and immediately all the doors were opened and everyone's chains were loosed.*

The world's people have prayed in churches, synagogues and places of worship and the Kingdom of Heaven has answered and given us

Ambush, the CURE for HIV/AIDS. For the body of Christ to receive it, we are still having some challenges.

A brief example is that of a 23 year old college student who contacted me saying that he was born with HIV, his biological father had long died and his mother was not doing so well and he wanted to know if Ambush was real and if I was speaking the truth. As we were talking, the Kingdom of Heaven gave me an open vision. I saw him in his room with brown carpet on the floor crying out to the Almighty for mercy. He was promising the LORD to do a certain thing that was between him and the LORD. I was then able to tell him the prayer he had made. He was shocked, frightened and surprised that I was able to give him such details. He then connected the conversation with his step father to hear what I was saying, but to our disappointment the man said that he does not believe anything I had said so the step son should not take Ambush because it was not true. I prayed for this young man because he had reached the stage there he had become resistant to three or four of the five types of ARV's and he was hoping that the researchers would find something new.

I could write volumes of these stories where the LORD gave me a 'word of knowledge' so specific to the individual that the only way I could know, I would have had to be there and I was not. The LORD has been doing this for many years so the people would know that I am speaking the truth. But somehow we have been trained to see first, then we believe where Jesus has it the right way which is to believe and you shall see.

Just like the prayers of Paul and Silas, hundreds of us have prayed and the prison chains of HIV have been broken for the millions of us who need and will need Ambush. Therefore the least we can do is to give thanks and praises to the MOST HIGH, JAHOVA, CREATOR of Heaven and Earth, for his grace, mercy and favor. Father, in the Mighty name of Jesus the Christ, we thank you for the gift of Ambush, we thank you for mercy, grace and favor in Jesus name. AMEN (readers kindly agree with me in prayer by saying aloud 'amen')

# HIV VACCINE......NOT POSSIBLE

A vaccine is a biological preparation that improves immunity to a particular disease. Vaccines usually contain a substance that resembles the disease causing microorganism and is often made from weakened or killed forms of the microbe. The substance stimulates the body's immune system to recognize the substance as an enemy, destroy it and remember the enemy so that the immune system can recognize and destroy any of the microorganisms it will encounter in the future.

If we had a vaccine for HIV today, how would it help the millions of people who are infected with HIV? The keepers of figures have been estimating that there are 30 to 40 million people who are infected for the past 10 years so who is really counting? Can they at this point? So do we blame the victims of alternate lifestyle? At the same time the world spends billions of its currencies in the search for a vaccine with no available solution.

As a health care practitioner, the more HIV spreads, the more dollars have to be spent. Here the drug companies, pharmacy owners or doctors will benefit from these dollars. There is nothing wrong with being a capitalist as a needed service is being provided but in the long run, the human society cannot afford the continuing drag of HIV/AIDS on its limited resources.

A few years ago I went for one of my usual 10 mile walks, in which there is a lot of time to talk to the Almighty. I asked the LORD,

"What about vaccine?" and He said,

"The testing of vaccines is like fist fighting your enemy for 28 years who has been beating you all along and now you give him a knife."

A vaccine for HIV is impossible because the LORD GOD JAHOVA has said so and His word is the law on earth. Then HIV is not homogenous because it was not created by the Creator but was probably made in a lab. Since every person represents a different 'strain' and there are almost 7 billion people on the planet, we would need that many vaccines which is also not possible. I use the word strain or type because HIV attaches to your DNA and since each person's DNA is different, then there is as many strains or types as there are people.

The possibilities of problems may be compounded if one thinks 'outside the box' to look at other animals. Is it possible that since HIV could have been made in a 'lab' and has crossed from other animals to man, that it could cross to all other warm blooded species? We have FIV or Feline AIDS in cats but the scientific community is quiet about dogs and we only hear of MERS or Middle Eastern Respiratory Syndrome when people start dying and it is postulated that maybe they contracted it from the camel. Did the camel get it from man?

The Kingdom of Heaven has said that since the virus has crossed from animal to man, then there is no barrier to infecting any or all warm blooded animals. To stop the spread of this disease, the Kingdom of Heaven has had to intervene because without such intervention, life as it is known would have been wiped off the face of the earth.

Ambush is therefore a gift, not only for use in man but in other animals so let us receive this gift with joy, gladness and thank the MOST HIGH JAHOVA for His goodness, grace, mercy and favor.

HIV/AIDS....The COST

There are many costs that are associated with HIV, such as the cost of drugs and treatments, the human cost and the social cost to the society or mankind. These costs may not have been incurred if there were no HIV, so how much better off would we have been without HIV?

The average cost of a triple drug tablet online for the treatment is advertised at $50 per tablet per day or $18, 250 per year or someone's salary. Monthly HIV treatments range from $2000 to $5000 with the major part going to pay for drugs. With life expectancy on the increase it is estimated to cost more than $500,000 per HIV infected person.

Let us look at a 20 year old who is infected and needs care at $20,000 to $25, 000 per year for the rest of his life. What about school? What about a career or training? Did he finish? Or even started? What about employment when he may be feeling sick most of the time? These questions are beginning to make me feel sick since there are no real answers but more questions.

We take this same 20 year old and what is his dream? It is hard to dream when you are not happy and not feeling well much more to do anything. This is a depressing scenario with a life doomed to sickness and despair no matter how well presented the advertisements are that claim that all you need to do is to take one pill a day and you will live a near normal life. At the same time you are cornered by stigma and no way of expressing how you are truly feeling.

If it costs half million to treat one HIV infected person and there is 1.1 million infected in the United States, then that is a large amount of money and growing because people are living longer and more people are being infected. Can the society afford it? Who is to pay this price tag for people who have not worked a day in their lives because of genuine illness? Can the society afford this cost with no prospect of getting a return on this investment? Any city administrator or politician grapples with these negative outflows while the ones left working are taxed to the max.

## COST....MY ONLY CHILD

To bring certain costs that are never put on paper with a dollar value, let me tell you a story. I spent a few years in Toronto, Canada while on this 'walk' with the LORD and gave Ambush to hundreds of people. At that time I had to prepare each batch of Ambush by boiling and giving the gallon of liquid.

There was this young man 20 years old, the only child of his middle aged mother. He was having chest pains since he was 15 years old and the doctors said he had a bad heart and so treated him for that complain and never checked to find the cause of a 20 year old on heart medications. His mother was at Church and was told by another lady who brought her son to me who was dying of AIDS, was treated with Ambush and he recovered.

Of hearing that there was a 'man of GOD', she brought the 20 year old to seek help from the LORD through me. He came to the house and was lugging an oxygen tank and its breathing apparatus. He was so weak and tired that he was not able to go up the 5 steps to the sitting area so I brought him a chair in the passageway and I sat in the steps. He was not interested in what I had to say at first, but the LORD gave me detailed specific instances of him having sex starting at age 14 or so. The LORD gave me such graphic details that he was compelled to listen and was very interested in knowing how I knew.

I told him that he had caught HIV and gave him a detailed description of the person who infected him. To this he agreed that I could not have known since I was not there so some force must be working for me to give him such details. He then agreed to take Ambush and I had very little supplies left at that time so I gave him the first dose and the gallon of Ambush. The LORD showed me that HIV caused his blood VOLUME to drop so the heart had to work twice as hard to circulate the half volume of blood. This is one of the reasons that the HIV infected experiences tiredness and difficulty climbing stairs.

While going home in the car, his mother questioned him as to what I said and he told her that I said he is infected with HIV. She had merely reached home when she called to tell me that all I had said to her only son was foolishness. He is only 20 and not a drug addict or a homosexual so he could not possible be infected so she is going to throw the Ambush away. I pleaded with her not to throw it away because I had a limited amount and more people who needed it. Then she hung up the phone in anger and disgust and threw the gallon of Ambush down the drain.

Fourteen days later, she buried her only son.

I was later told that she was just asking one question, "What would have happened if she had allowed him to drink the Ambush?"

When ever the LORD does anything He always says what he is going to do before he does it so that when it comes to fruition, He gets all the praise and the glory. In Joshua 6:2 the LORD said to Joshua,

*"See! I have given Jericho into your hands, its kings and the mighty men of valor"*.

At this time the battle was not yet fought, but the LORD who knows the end before the fight has started and could say who would win. In the case of Ambush, the Angel said he is giving me the CURE for HIV/AIDS, so he who has supernatural powers has brought us HOPE. We need to believe that it will work but over the years and the hundreds who have taken Ambush, we have seen it work so we can give thanks and praise for what

the Kingdom of Heaven has given ALL
OF US. Thank you Jesus!!

HIV ..........PREVENTION

The World is now gearing its people towards prevention which indicates a partial failure to find a cure or a vaccine. This is good, honorable and a pleasing move to those who are not yet infected. But what about the 30 to 50 million who are infected? Or those who do not yet know they are infected since there is a window period for the seroconversion?

There is a law or recognized rule in virology that when a case of epidemiologic infection presents itself as a clinical manifestation of a disease, then there are 99 subclinical cases coming or in the pipelines. This is a calculation of the number of persons that an individual interacts or comes in contact with within the period of time for the disease to manifest. HIV may take up to 7 years before the there are clinical symptoms. If we in the United States have 1.1 million infected with HIV, then we can expect 110 million subclinical cases on infection in the pipeline. Is this a good time to start prevention or has the horse left the barn and we are merely closing an empty barn?

Condoms

We are told to wrap ourselves in condoms which is a good idea when it comes to unwanted pregnancies but how well does it work for the virus. On research one may find that there are natural holes in the latex condom of about 5 microns and a sperm is about 1 micron. So the condom works in blocking sperm cells. The size of the HIV virus is 0.1 micron and the size of the condom holes still remain at 5 microns. Do we need a rocket scientist to tell us that it is possible that the virus may pass through the condom?

Saliva

There are many sources that say HIV may not be transmitted by saliva. If that is the case then why are HIV infected persons who spit at officers charged with assault with a deadly weapon or worst, charged as a bio-terrorist? Then if it were a public fact that HIV may be transmitted by saliva, this would further alienate the infected. More scorn might be exhibited by those who are not HIV positive so it might be a political ploy to keep saying it is might not be possible. I was grappling with this issue the LORD again showed me otherwise.

One Saturday I visited a synagogue in Miami for the second time. It was a small congregation of about 20 attending that Sabbath. There I met a gentleman of about 55 years old and he was accompanied by his only child, a 5 year old son. This was the first time meeting and we started talking and he realized that I am a Pharmacist so he started to tell me that his son Ryan has never been out of an ear infection for the last year or so. He declared that the right ear would be infected, he takes Ryan to the pediatrician, get some pink medicine which may be assumed to be amoxicillin, the ear would clear up in the week and the following week the child would have an infection in the left ear and he was back to the doctor's office. He was clearly disturbed and while speaking the LORD showed me in an open vision, meaning I am awake, what the problem was.

I was taken in the 'Spirit' to Ryan's daycare where there were a number of brightly colored balls about 2-3 inches in diameter and they were coated with different flavor smelling paints, such as strawberry or orange depending on the color balls. The tendencies were that the kids would suck on these balls and the room had 15 to 20 kids. The LORD showed me that was the method by which Ryan had contracted HIV even though both his parents are HIV negative. When the

LORD gives a word of knowledge, He does not give it so we can say we knew, but that some changes to others may ensue.

Here is this man with his only son of 5 years old to be told that he is HIV positive was a terrible notion to me so I decided to leave the service before it was finished so I would not have to say anything to the man. So before the last prayer, I got up and walked out into the dining area so I could sneak out unnoticed but there was Ryan. He grabbed on my leg and would not let go as if his life depended on it. Later his father came out and apologized that it was the first time Ryan had done such a thing. I confessed that the child was right and I was wrong in trying to leave with the word of the LORD.

I then explained the vision I had seen and told him to ask the pediatrician to order a Western blot test so he would at least start the talks on what that test was for and the conversation about HIV would begin.

Working in the hospital I noticed a lot of human growth hormones being prescribed for patients whose profile resembles that of an HIV positive person since certain thing were not documented if you were a rich paying customer. The rules are different for the poor or Medicaid/Medicare paying patient. On further research, human growth hormone is an anabolic steroid which grows muscles and decrease the wasting syndrome associated with HIV.  So these agents are used to ward off some of the unwanted effects of HIV.

I asked the LORD why the kids with HIV do not readily get sick and He explained that the kids are growing and have an ample supply of natural human growth hormones. Theses substances are able to keep the virus in check and keep the kids healthy for the most part.

Kids that do get sick sometimes have cuts, sores or an athletic kid might injure a muscle which gives place for the virus to form pockets but they will get sick in general when they have stopped growing. At the age of 19 or 20 when the growth hormones decrease, then the virus balloons or explodes and the battle begins.

I was contacted by a 19 year old from Georgia, who works at a fast food restaurant that he was HIV positive and was having all the symptoms and had gone to the free clinic for the diarrhea he was having. He was ordered some antidiarrheal medicine and sent home. The diarrhea did not subside and he claims to be losing weight very fast. I sent him Ambush and by the third day the diarrhea stopped. I did not hear from him for 2 weeks and I called to see how he was doing. He said his mother threw away the Ambush that it is foolishness. A month later, the mother called me to say her son was vey sick and having severe headaches, fever and that there was no relief from the clinic and asked if there was there anything I could suggest.

We are hurt so badly by our unbelief or the programming by national sources that if it not on the TV, it is bad and wrong. What method would we like to receive from the ALMIGHTY? How should he send HOPE? If it is not coming from the scientific community who are not in tune to the knowledge of the Almighty, then it is rejected. It makes me wonder how many of the answers to mans' problems are in the bodies of those who have died? If I were to die now, how would we get the answer that we have been praying for? Would one of those who got the benefit of Ambush ever talk?

Matthew 5: 14-16 Jesus speaking says,

*"You are the light of the World, a city that is set on a hill cannot be*

*hidden, nor do they light a lamp and put it under a basket, but on a lamp stand and it gives light to all who are in the house. Let your light so shine before men that they may see your good works and glorify your Father in Heaven."*

The word light means knowledge as in revelation knowledge from the Kingdom of Heaven given for the benefit on the Earth. The thinkers of today see the eureka moment as the aha! moment and they think it just popped into their heads. This thought or bright idea, had to come from somewhere, and if it did, then how can we have a continuous flow of these ideas?

The answer is simply put that the Kingdom of Heaven through the Holy Spirit gives these moments and they can be continuous if you are working on one of His projects on earth. It also takes time, patience and perseverance to listen to the voice of the ALMIGHTY, and OBEY what he has commanded. Too often we hear the voice but refuse to obey so He does not speak so loudly after that and lots of revelation is lost.

Therefore we give the LORD all the praise and the glory for giving us Ambush, the CURE for HIV/AIDS and although it has not yet come to fruition, it gives HOPE to the millions infected and ALL OF US.

## THE OWNER of AMBUSH

Ambush does not belong to Apostle Shada Mishe, and was not given to me for me but to ALL OF US. Psalm 29:10 says

*The LORD is KING forever*

Since the LORD is a King, He picks whom he chooses to give his commands to, and He does not pick a committee but one man to do the job. So in June of 2007, He commanded me to file a patent on Ambush which was filed on June 21, 2007. A registered patent application was filed with the United States Patent and Trademark Office in Alexandria, Virginia

Appl ication # US     11/820,540

Filing date              6/21/2007

| | |
|---|---|
| Art unit | 1614 |
| Filing fee rec'd | $500 |
| Total claims | 11 |
| Ind. Claims | 3 |
| Confirmation # | 3585 |
| Owner of Patent | Jewish State of Israel |
| Worker | Apostle Shada Mishe |

We will all benefit from this gift to ALL OF US, but the owner is the Jewish State of Israel. The Angel said it is to be free to the people but Israel is to industrially produce Ambush and sell to the Worlds' governments which will give it free to their people.

In 2009, I was in Toronto, Canada as part of the training process when the LORD said to me,

"Go to the Israeli Embassy in Toronto and give then Ambush"

So I went to the Embassy and spoke to someone behind a dark glass and told the person that the LORD GOD of Abraham, Isaac and Jacob gave me Ambush, the CURE for HIV/AIDS and I was to give it to them. The person behind the glass said they have nothing to do with anything concerning HIV and did not know what I was talking about.

I told her to write down what I had said for a future date since I had to fill out a form with my name, address, telephone and nature of business. So I left the embassy and went home. As I walked through the door, the phone rang and it was the same lady from the embassy asking me to repeat my nature of business, of which I repeated what the LORD had told me to tell them.

I can now publicly write that I have given Ambush over to the Jewish State of Israel as a gift from the LORD JESUS the Christ and with further instruction to be delivered at the appropriate time.

In the First Book of Samuel, chapter 1, Hannah prayed for a male child and promised to give him give him back to the LORD all the days of his life. Her request was granted and she presented Samuel, the young child back to the LORD.

In our case, the Body of Christ prayed for the CURE for HIV/AIDs for many years. Our petition has been granted, and I was privileged to be chosen to present it back to the LORD

for His use on the Earth. Therefore
we raise our voices in praises,
thanksgiving and worship to the KING
of KINGS and LORD of LORDS, the
MOST HIGH JAHOVA for all his
goodness, mercy, grace and favor.

## SEROREVERSION

SERO- CONVERSION of HIV is the time in which a person develops antibodies for HIV but does not yet test positive on the HIV antibody test. This means it is the time that the body changes from HIV antibody negative to HIV antibody positive. The time for this change over is called the window period.

In the early days of giving Ambush I understood the virological principle that once the body came into contact with a virus, then antibodies would be formed and person would be HIV positive for life. I was so WRONG!, but that was what I studied in schools and what I had heard said in the HIV lectures and continuing education credits that I took for a number of years, so I was sure they are all correct. But I was so WRONG!!!!

On February 16, 2012, I had a vision and the Kingdom of Heaven said to me

'S E R O R E V E R S I O N'

So I got up and wrote it down because it was clearly spelt to me more than once and very slowly. In the morning I remembered that I had gotten a word of knowledge and it said 'seroreversion' so I put it down thinking that there were no such words and the Kingdom may have gotten it wrong and I reasoned my self out of the word. There was a tug on my spirit the following day to look up the word. Lo and behold it meant the opposite of seroconversion, which is the time the tests can no longer detect antibodies in the persons' bodies. Then I remembered that a number of people who had taken Ambush were now testing HIV negative.

The first person to report that she had now tested negative was Miss Washington DC. I met her on H Street in DC in the hot month of August 2007. She approached me and asked me if I wanted to be tested for HIV. I said no because the LORD had given me the CURE for HIV. I was at the same time handing out fliers to say that Ambush CURES HIV/AIDS and recruiting takers. She quickly said that she was a child of GOD and could feel the anointing on me so she agreed to take it. I went home, prepared the Ambush and took it to her house and she gulped down the first dose straight from the bottle. In January I left DC but kept in touch by Facebook.

In the spring of 2008, I was in Toronto and she emailed me that she was now testing negative, I was more than elated so I called for verbal conformation which I got. Then I asked her if she was going to go public with what had happened. She said no and that the LORD would bring Ambush to fruition real soon.  I still send her emails to check on her status and all seems well since she had made a vow never to have sex again if she was ever cured of the disease.

I have spoken of one person, but the LORD has said that by the mouth of 2 or 3 witnesses a thing shall be established. So I was on the look out for others.

The second person to serorevert to being HIV negative was Pastor Pretoria. He was a 24 year old pastor in Pretoria who saw where I would paste on the internet at the bottom of articles, in the comment section that Ambush CURES HIV/AIDS. So he contacted me by email to say he was HIV positive and very depressed and distraught because he found that he was HIV positive and went to his Bishop for counseling and solace. The Bishop said to him,

"You have just finished your seminary in time to go to the cemetery"

These words were more destructive that the disease, but I could not send him Ambush because I was only taught to prepare the liquid and it was not going to be possible to send the gallon from Toronto to South Africa without it spoiling and a high cost of postage which I did not have. This was in late 2009 so it bothered my spirit and the Kingdom of Heaven gave me a word of knowledge in earl y 2010 as how to select a piece of the dried wood, grind it and send it in a bubble pack envelope. I was so excited and on February 20, 2010 I mailed him Ambush and the preparation instruction. His words of reply were,

"I believe that if this works, then we can help a very great number of people, to help in churches and beyond. I am standing by waiting for it"

He emailed me every day for the next two weeks for solace and assurance that it would work. He received the package two weeks later and sent me pictures of him preparing the Ambush. He consumed the first batch and complained that he was having skin problems of itching so I told him to use peanut oil to rub the rashes and to make sure I sent him another pack of Ambush.

Six months later he found a lady to marry and he went with her to check her status and while he was there, she pressed him check his.

Lo and behold, his came back HIV negative, so he emailed me with his great news. I then asked him to send me a copy of both his positive and his negative and that was never done. Slowly he stopped emailing me and I would send an email and he might answer in 2 weeks until he has stopped answering. I have given his email address to a number of people and told then that he has seen Ambush work but he has never answered any of them.

But thanks be to GOD I still have emails where he said he had tested HIV negative and his pictures on line shows a healthy looking pastor who now conducts the funerals for his dead parishioners.

We have had two witnesses so far, but The LORD has given me three for this book and the third in the story of Mr. Cleveland and Miss Ohio on the USA. In August of 2012, Miss

Ohio emailed me that Mr. Cleveland was just tested and was found to be HIV positive and the Clinic had requested that she presents herself for testing at the earliest convenient date. She was very depressed and wished to speak with me so I gave her my number and we began talking. I learnt that she had 5 kids, it is the heights of Summer and her electricity had been turned off. The LORD said I was to pay her bill which I did and sent her 2 packs of Ambush.

I explained to her that they were both to take Ambush at the same time and she was not to go to get tested until she had finished Ambush and waited for 5 months. I had learnt that if the window period is about 3 months for seroconversion, then it should take the same time to serorevert and I had seen where HIV positive people who went to the SCOAN (Synagogue Church of All Nations) in Lagos, Nigeria and were healed of HIV, they would become HIV negative in about 5 months.

They both took Ambush at the same time and one of its effects or side effect if the increase in libido which has produced child number 6.

Miss Ohio waited exactly 5 months and got tested at the County Clinic and behold, she was HIV negative. On the other side Mr. Cleveland was pressed to go and get retested but he refused but in August of 2013, he was arrested and put in the County Jail. There he only spent 4 days and was tested for HIV. He was told that he is HIV negative at the time of testing. Now he is more than happy because both he and his lady are HIV negative.

Then the LORD said to me that I was to tell him to go back to the County jail and ask for a record that he was tested 4 days ago. They are compelled by law to give him a copy then he is to take both pieces of paper to the local newspaper and share his story and he would receive two million dollars ($2,000,000) when he has finished his speaking engagements. I told him a number of times and he always said he was going to do it but never did.

In January of 2014 he finally went to the Jail where he was tested negative for a copy of his results. The jail staff told him that there was no record of him in the computer but were willing to test him again. This time they drew a few vials of blood and told him to come back the next day. Then the staff told him that there is something wrong with his blood and they cannot read his test so they need to take some more blood. He allowed then to take a second sample of blood in February and again he was told that they "cannot read his results because there is something wrong with his blood".

In April 2014 he was picked up for a parole violation and placed in jail. He was then transferred to the HIV section because his former HIV test had resurfaced saying that he is HIV positive. Had he listened and obeyed the words and instructions of the LORD and gone back to the Jail on day 5 to retrieve his negative paper, would things have been different? If he is truly negative will the truth be told?

There are many others who after having received Ambush and promised to go public with their results have gone silent and their contacts cold to dead. But I did not start this project, it does not belong to me and according to Philippians 1: 6,

*"being confident of this very thing , that he who has begun a good work in you will complete it until the day of Jesus Christ."*

Since Ambush was started by the Kingdom of Heaven when an Angel was sent to give me the CURE for HIV/AIDS and not by Apostle Shada Mishe, then the Kingdom of

Heaven will finish what they started so there is HOPE that Ambush will come to fruition and HOPE for the millions who are infected, affected and ALL OF US.

I was ordered by the Almighty to send a copy of the 28 minute video that is presently on Youtube to the 70 biggest and most influential Church bodies in the United States and to my shock, not a single one answered my letter that accompanied the video.

The LORD wants Ambush to come to fruition through the body of Christ. His intention was that the Church with theirs elders who have the Spirit of Discernment would have listened to the video and would discern whether I was speaking the truth or not. Finding that I am speaking the truth, they would get a supply of Ambush for their sick HIV positive end stage or ARV's resistant members and watch the LORD work.

The LORD works by faith and faith is the substance HOPED for, which in this case is the CURE for HIV/AIDS. Who better is there to give than the people who prayed for the CURE? No body or group of people that the LORD has sent me to so far has accepted anything I have said and I know that I speak the truth and yet the body of Christ treat me with such disdain and as if I am 'crazy'. I have been doing what He has ordered for the last 12 years and there is no reason for me to stop now or worst to turn back and reject the Almighty because a few people has rejected me.

## THE KINGDOM OF HEAVEN

In 1953, I was born in Jamaica which was a colony of Great Britain or United Kingdom. I was taught from childhood to always say 'God save the queen'. This is because in 1952, Queen Elizabeth II was made Queen over Great Britain and her colonies which included Canada, Australia and Jamaica to name a few. The Queen was head over Great Britain and also head of the Jamaican government. Her representative in Jamaica was the Governor who was the Queens' mouthpiece who spoke the intent and desires of her. In Jamaica we were taught the culture of Great Britain, eat with a knife and fork, drink tea at 6pm, dressed like the British, spoke the Queen's English and the culture of the UK came to Jamaica.

All the land in Jamaica were owned by the Queen and the people were citizens of Great Britain and had British passports. The Kingdom of Great Britain in a sense came to Jamaica. So the standard of life was made to resemble that of a citizen who was living in Britain. If we in Jamaica were hungry or needed shelter we called on the Queen, through her Governor. It would be disgraceful on the part of the Queen if her subjects were in need and she could not attend to them since she was the sole owner of all the lands and all the people.

The Queen spoke very timely and precisely because her words were the Law of not only Britain but all the countries or Commonwealth under her. Since she owned everything, then her wealth was common to all and she could not be voted out because she was not voted in and was there for life.

In a Democracy, the president is not in the position for life, does not own the lands or the people and can be impeached before his term has ended. The body of Christ in the western world thinks that the Queen is the head, similar to the President being the head and there is really no difference. This is a wrong idea of kingdom principles and so there are challenges in understanding the Kingdom of Heaven.

The Epistle of Paul the Apostle to the Galatians Chapter 4: 4 says,

*But when the fullness or time had come, God sent forth his Son born of a woman, born under the law.*

The fullness of time or the right time was that Jesus the Christ was sent when there was a type of government on earth that mirrored the one in Heaven. Jesus was born when Herod was king who sent soldiers to kill the young children in Bethlehem at his word, no Congress, no committee. When Jesus was crucified the Governor was Pilate in Jerusalem and the King was Caesar in Rome. So when Jesus explained the Kingdom of Heaven, the people could understand because they were living in the Kingdom of Caesar.

Today, the Kingdom of Heaven is here on Earth and the Governor or mouthpiece for Heaven is here as the

Holy Spirit. He is the invisible communicator between the invisible Kingdom of Heaven and the visible Kingdom on men. In the Jamaican example, we lived in Jamaica but we were in the Kingdom of Great Britain. We therefore live in two worlds in the visible Kingdom of Earth and the invisible Kingdom of Heaven when we believe that GOD exists and believe in Him. Heaven has communicated with Earth and given us AMBUSH which now gives HOPE to the millions of infected and affected people.

AMBUSH    THE MESSAGE

YOU MUST BELIEVE THAT HE
EXISTS

Let us start from the beginning
of The Book, The BIBLE, on day one,
page one and line one says "in the
beginning GOD." There must have
been a beginning and we are in the
middle so there must be an end.
Man cannot explain how, what,
where and why we are here or how
we as humans came into being. The
Creator of all that is seen and
unseen knows perfectly well what
was, what is and what will be. Every
manufacturer of a product prints an
instruction booklet as how to use
the product and get the best results.
If you purchased a car, the
manufacture will tell you to put a
certain grade gasoline in the gas

tank. Now since the car belongs to you, you have all rights of putting anything in the gas tank including milk or water and see if the car runs.

In the same way, man was created by the LORD GOD JAHOVA and he used chosen or anointed men on earth to write the instruction manual called THE BIBLE. Like the owner of the car, man was given the will of choice. He can choose to read the instructions and abide by then or do what ever 'feels good" to him, but like the car, if you put water in the gas tank it will not start.

There are times when there is a defect and the manufacturer recalls the cars to fix the defect. He is not merely asking you to bring in the car to change the braking system but you are compelled to bring it in for replacement or risk having no brakes and ending up in a ditch. You have a choice so you take in the car. Right? Right! Because you believe that the manufacturer will restore the braking system to the original or intended condition.

If you can believe that the manufacturer will do what he has said he will do and has the ability to do it, why is it so hard for humans to believe that he was created by the Creator? There are so many monkey stories as to how man came into being without reading the instruction manual of mankind. We men are good at trying to fit up a piece of furniture from what we "feel", only to resort to the instruction manual in frustration when what we feel does not work. For 30 to 40 years we have been fighting with the disease HIV and it is time to go back to the manufacturer or Creator for answers, but first we must believe that He exists.

The instruction manual of mankind otherwise known as The Bible in the Book of Hebrews chapter 11:6 says,

*But without faith it is impossible to please Him, for he who comes to GOD must believe that He is, and that He is a rewarder of those who diligently seek him.*

If you believe that the manufacturer can and will fix the car, then by that same belief that you must, you have to, you are compelled to believe that the Creator exists. You have no choice but to face the consequence if you refuse. The LORD GOD JAHOVA is a great King and what he says is the Law from the invisible Kingdom of Heaven to the visible Kingdom of men on the Earth. Believers have been praying for years for relief from HIV/AIDS and they are then compelled to believe that The LORD gives reward for their diligence to which He has given us Ambush, the CURE for HIV/AIDS.

Is it possible for a Pharmacist working two full time jobs to think all these things by himself? How would he know which plant to pick? Could he guess the dose? Why has it worked? While the scientific research community have drawn blanks all these years? The answer is that some other source must be supplying him with the knowledge. These words that he has received could only come from the Creator, which it has. Thank you Creator! You have given us HOPE. Thank you.

## YOU ARE COMPELLED TO COME IN

The second part of Ambush the Message, is that first you have been compelled to believe that the LORD GOD JAHOVE exists, now you are being compelled to believe in Him. In my early years of listening to the Almighty, I was in Central Florida one Sunday morning and had three hours from 9 to 12 to spare so I decided to go to the nearest church. I asked the receptionist at the hotel and she directed me to drive one block and make a left and there is the Church. I followed the directions but did not see a church so I kept driving for the next 30 minutes when I spotted a Methodist Church and people were gathering so I went there. In that church the Pastor read Luke 14:33 which says,

*Then the master said to the servant, "Go out into the highways and hedges and compel them to come in that my house may be filled."*

When I heard the words 'compel them' I was immediately taken up in the Spirit into a different realm where the words were burnt into my spirit and I was asking the LORD if the end was really near. More needs to be done to compel unbelievers to come to The LORD GOD JAHOVA through Jesus the Christ.

We know from research that HIV kills brain cells and with it, memory loss because the brain has similar features to a computer. If you have information in a file and the computer crashes, then you loose that file. If you put that file on an external source such as a disc and the computer crashes you may be able to retrieve form the disc. If one of the operating systems is lost then you have to go to the manufacturer for restoration.

HIV causes memory loss which is one of the operating systems and the only way to receive restoration is to go to the manufacturer, The LORD GOD JAHOVA. In his storeroom, he has the most updated memory system in Jesus the Christ. You are therefore compelled to believe in him or go to him for mental restoration.

The gift of Ambush the drug that kills the virus that causes AIDS is proof that the LORD GOD JAHOVA,

Maker of Heaven and Earth exists, or how else would we have gotten it? It also says that to receive certain benefits such as the healing of the brain by restoration of memory, you are compelled to believe in Him.

## THANKS AND PRAISE

How do you thank some one who has first given you the gift of life? Then the Evil one whose only purpose is to kill, steal and destroy has given you HIV? He has stolen your joy because you might pretend you are happy, but you are not. You are compelled to live in a state of sickness for the rest of your life and know that the older you get, the more illnesses are poured out unto you and the more you have to muster inner strength to live one day at a time. You are compelled to take daily medications if you are fortunate. In poor countries, you are not given ARV's until you are close to dying so a lot has been stolen from you.

HIV has destroyed millions of lives due to illness. You could not finish school so now you cannot get or hold a job. If you had a job and it was known by your employers, they might fire you. Your spouse or partner finding that you are HIV positive while they are still negative might decide to leave town. These are lives destroyed by HIV because the dreams will never be fulfilled and all you are able to HOPE for is a quick and painless end.

Then the Evil one will kill all those who are infected with HIV. It may not be today but it is sure to come before the natural span of time. So he gets the last laugh after punishing you for years, then you die a miserable death with sores and diarrhea and the worst for some is an intact mind that now turns against you and there is nothing that you can do.

We now turn to the parents and caregivers and as a parent, when I bury my children, who is left to bury me? Who will carry on the family? We look at the caregivers who have caught HIV themselves in the process and I can still hear this young caregiver who after drawing blood from a HIV positive patient, accidentally stuck herself with the same needle and said,

"Lord, he killed me!"

Was it worth going to work that day? What about her family and friends? And the web and vicious cycle of killing, stealing and destruction continues. Where is the HOPE? Where can we turn for help? The help can only come from the invisible Kingdom of Heaven, here on earth through the Holy Spirit.

We have prayed for years for relief from the burden of HIV/AIDS and the Kingdom of Heaven has heard our prayers and has given us Ambush, the CURE for HIV/AIDS. The method or packaging for delivery may not have been what we were expecting, but let us join hands and hearts and give thanks, praise and glory to the KING of Kings and LORD of Lords, the LORD GOD JAHOVA.

I pray a prayer of thanksgiving for the wonderful gift that we have received on behalf of ALL OF US  as found in 1 Chronicles 16:8-9

*Oh give thanks to the LORD!*

*Call upon his name:*

*Make known his deeds among the peoples:*

*Sing to Him, sing psalms to Him:*

*Talk of all His wondrous works!*

Or in Psalm 136:1-4

*Oh, give thanks to the LORD, for He is good!*

*For His mercy endures forever.*

*Oh, give thanks to the GOD of gods!*

*For His mercy endures forever.*

*Oh, give thanks to the LORD of lords!*

*For His mercy endures forever.*

*To Him who alone does great wonders,*

*For his mercy endures forever.*

AMEN.

www.ingramcontent.com/pod-product-compliance
Lightning Source LLC
Chambersburg PA
CBHW072026190526
45166CB00015B/516